How to Lower Blood Pressure Naturally & Quickly

Powerful Tricks to Deal with Hypertension Using Supplements and Other Natural Remedies

By

Kim Hilton

Table of Contents

Introduction

As blood flows through the artery, stress is exerted against the walls. This stress is referred to blood pressure. Hypertension is synonymous to blood pressure, and there is an increased number of people suffering from hypertension in America and around the world each year. Although the occurrence of high blood pressure is more common among adults, recent common cases have been discovered even among young adults. High blood pressure itself doesn't have a direct symptom but makes the body vulnerable to health problems and ailments which could be life-threatening. These health problems might include kidney diseases, stroke, vision loss, and heart failure. It is very important to take all necessary steps in lowering blood pressure in order to maintain good health and energy.

This book is focused on natural ways you can lower blood pressure without spending a lot, and in the process cultivating better attitude for good health. The strategies are focused on stimulating your immunity and providing a backbone to circumvent the occurrence of any ailment relating to high blood pressure.

CHAPTER 1: Causes of High Blood Pressure

Pregnancy

Pregnant women are more vulnerable to high blood pressure compared to their counterparts.

Psoriasis

Diabetes and high blood pressure are also connected to psoriasis. It shows as scaly patches, red and thick on the skin. It appears gradually and gets worst when left untreated.

Diabetes

The high sugar content of the blood normally referred to as type 1 diabetes increases the risk of developing hypertension unless due treatment practices are being administered and implemented.

Mental stress

Mental stress is one of the commonest causes of hypertension. Long-term stress, especially from worries, tends to control the air traffic and ultimately causes mental stress in the end.

High-fat diet

Diet with a high level of fat content tends to expose the body to the risk of developing high blood pressure. Also, the type and sources of fat determine the level of vulnerability for high blood pressure. Better sources of fats include the omega oils, olive oil, nuts, and avocados.

Alcohol intake

Alcohol intake is related to mental stress, and on the other hand, exposes the body to the risk of developing systolic blood pressure.

Smoking

The narrowing of blood vessels is caused by smoking, which ultimately leads to high blood pressure. This occurs when the amount of blood that has to flow to the heart is being reduced, therefore causing faster heart rate.

Physical inactivity

Inactive people are at more risk of developing high blood pressure than people who perform exercises on a daily basis.

Gender

At all ages, blood pressure is common among men than women, even though at older ages this rate tends to equal.

Obesity

Obesity is related to high fat and sedentary lifestyle. High blood pressure is among the ailments the overweight individuals are at high risk of developing.

Background

Unlike the Amerindians or Caucasians, researches have indicated that "people from the South Asian and African ethnic background are at greater risk of developing high blood pressure."

Temperature

In times of higher temperatures, high blood pressure cases tend to be lower, and highest cases in the period of lower temperatures. Ultimately cold contributes to the development of diastolic and systolic blood pressure.

Family history

A person is more likely to develop high blood pressure when there is a history of hypertension on the family. This doesn't mean that you must develop high blood pressure if your parents have it.

Age

Apparently, older people are at more risk of developing high blood pressure. This is because of the factors of an exhausted body system, mental stress and other ailments related to old age.

CHAPTER 2:Signs and Symptoms of High Blood Pressure

Breathlessness

Palpitations

Nosebleeds

Double vision

Blurred vision

Dizziness

Vomiting

Nausea

Headache

CHAPTER 3:
Complications Caused by High Blood Pressure

Retarded brain functions

Memory or recalling problems

Metabolic syndrome

Torn eye blood vessels

Kidney disease

Aneurysm

Blood clotting

Heart failure

Heart attack

Stroke

CHAPTER 4: Ways to Lower Your Blood Pressure

Cut down on caffeine

According to the body system, the consistent intake of caffeine stimulates blood pressure and exposes you to ailments related to hypertension. The first good step to take is to cut down on caffeine by taking decaffeinated energy drinks and coffee. If you are a coffee lover, it is only better to look for alternatives such as green tea.

Drink less alcohol

Alcohol is one of the greatest catalysts for blood pressure. Every 35 ounces of alcohol you put into your body raises 1mmHg of your blood pressure. Moderate drinking is emphasized but cutting back completely from alcohol might not be a good idea. The aim is to lower your blood pressure, and so you are required to watch what you put into your body.

Consider Blood Pressure Lowering Supplements

Blood pressure lowering supplements such as magnesium, whey protein, and omega-3 are effective in lowering the blood pressure to a significant level. Since high blood pressure is also related to magnesium deficiency, patients have used magnesium supplements for the purpose of lowering blood pressure. Whey protein is derived from milk, and it has always been confirmed to lower blood pressure.

Omega 3, on the other hand, is a polyunsaturated fatty acid often gotten in fish oil and works best in lowering pressure especially when consumed regularly.

Consider High Protein Foods

People that consume high protein foods are less vulnerable to diseases which also includes high blood pressure. They have a very active immunity, and their body is well-balanced to regularize stress and other physical alterations that contribute to the rise in blood pressure. One hundred grams of protein consumed daily will drastically bring down the risk of developing high blood pressure to 40 percent. Foods that contain high protein include:

Cheese

Chickpeas

Nuts

Beans

Beans

Poultry

Eggs

Fish

Consume More Garlic

Garlic has also been proved to have qualities needed to lower blood pressure. Preferably, garlic extract when included in meals or taken regularly will help reduce the risk of developing high blood pressure or hypertension. Studies have shown that garlic should come first when it comes to the natural consumable foods to be recommended for lowering of blood pressure.

Sleep More

Even though sleep is considered among the causes of obesity, another research has found out that an increase in the number of sleeping hours could reduce the level of blood pressure significantly.

The aim is to have an undisturbed night sleep and also to get at least 20-minutes nap in the afternoon.

Sleeping is the best way to reduce stress and ultimately helps in activating the immune system, making sure you become less vulnerable to the things that may elevate the blood pressure.

Use Medicinal Herbs

Herbs also work the magic in lowering blood pressure. All that matter is choosing the kinds of herbs you can get access to, and you are also comfortable with. Most modern medications for blood pressure are originated from herbs but in a reduced form. It is necessary that you take the natural form of the medication in order to feel well again.

These herbs may include:

Umbrella tree bark

Oolong tea

Green tea

Tomato extract

Sesame oil

Roselle

River Lily

Maritime pine bark

Indian Plantago

Giant dodder

Ginger root

Coffee weed

Chinese hawthorn

Celery juice

Cat's clay

And black bean.

Do not take herbal supplements without the supervision of a pharmacist or a healthcare provider. Always make sure you are on the safer side especially when you are on prescriptions. Prescription medications might interfere with the effectiveness of the herb.

Consume Dark Chocolate

Cacao chocolate is highly recommended for the effective lowering of blood pressure. The Harvard Medical School study has confirmed this. Unsweetened chocolates, which contain flavonoids help the dilation of the blood vessels. Make sure that you consume the ones without sugar, most common in dark chocolate. It is necessary that you take the chocolate daily in order to provide for the widening of the blood vessels consistently.

Yoga or Meditation

Yoga provides for mindfulness, which is a great element for meditation. Mindfulness gives total control over stress and occurrences that might stimulate the emotions causing even more stress. It provides for attentiveness and controlled impulsivity when it comes to thinking and a whole decision-making mindset of an individual.

In blood pressure, the magical effect of mindful meditation is through a drastic reduction in stress. Experiments to prove the theory of mindfulness has found out that mindfulness can lower blood pressure with around four mmHg.

Reduce Stress

Specifically, work on several tactics available to help you reduce stress. You don't have to keep working if you don't have to. Allow time for stillness, where you don't have to do anything. In stillness, you are not even required to think. Just sit in a quiet place and let things roll naturally.

You might have a family and workplace demands tied on your neck, but you have to allow time for your person, to revamp and reload. The first way to reduce stress is by cutting back on things that cause stress. Stop doing things when you don't have to do them, and only focus on necessities. Learn to delegate at home and in the office.

Listen to good music, watch comedy, take a walk and practice deep breathing in order to relieve stress. You will find yourself worrying less and doing more things that will contribute to your happiness and satisfaction.

Stop Smoking

Regardless of how hard, you have to take the brave step of cutting back completely from smoking. If you can't do it on your own, then it is an addiction, and you might need some help. Join support groups or/and start seeing a counselor, where you will talk about options and motivations for stopping.

Smoking ultimately increases the heart rate and therefore forcing stress. On the other hand, "the tobacco chemicals may cause significant damage to the blood vessels, making the arteries to narrow."

Cut Back On Processed Foods

Processed foods contain extra everything. Extra sugar, extra salt, and even extra fat. Chemicals found in processed foods are overwhelmingly dangerous to your general wellbeing. And in your attempt to lower your blood pressure, you have to cut back almost completely on processed foods. You have to give up on all the snacks, chips, pizza, canned soups, and deli meats. Only consume fast foods and snacks with low sodium, specifically below 5.

Consume More Potassium

Even as you consume less sodium, it is only advisable to take more potassium. Potassium is one of the most important food elements also useful for lowering blood pressure. Specifically, potassium disarms the negative effects of excessive salt consumption.

Natural sources of potassium are often recommended in order to avoid other chemicals:

Vegetables such as spinach, greens, tomato, potato, sweet potato, etc., are good sources of potassium to be considered.

Fruits such as oranges, apricots, and banana also contain a good deal of potassium, especially banana.

Fish

Dairy foods.

Cut Down On Sugar

Refined carbohydrate and sugar work hand in hand. Individuals wanting to lose some pounds are best advised to cut down on refined carbohydrates and sugar, so also on the course of lowering blood pressure.

Go for low-carb diet consistently in order to lower your blood pressure. Instead of cutting down on sugar, replace your habits with a healthy low-carb diet to improve your health. Not just blood pressure, low-carb diet also helps in reducing the risk of heart disease.

Lose Weight

There are different methods of losing weight that are healthy and fast. All you have to keep in mind is your objective: to lower your blood pressure. Other medical problems can also be averted by simply losing 10 pounds more.

Exercise More

Exercise is not just about going to the gym or being monitored while performing some crunches. Exercise might just mean taking a walk around your house. It could mean trekking to your workplace instead of taking the bus or going with your car.

It could also mean going to the gym and spending some 20 minutes. Jogging, walking, sports, etc., are all parts of exercise that you can be implemented according to how comfortable you are with a particular practice.

Exercises help the heart to become stronger. As a result, it pumps blood in and out with lesser efforts, putting less pressure on the arteries. Less pressure on the arteries always means a lowered blood pressure.

CHAPTER 5:
Natural/Holistic Practices in the Treatment of High Blood Pressure

In natural healing, there are certain ways we treat high blood **pressure.**

1. Herbalism

This is the most popular part of natural treatments. There are hundreds of herbs that have been used and are still being used to treat high blood pressure.

Herbalism can be approached in two different ways. The use of Herbs and correcting bad nutrition while promoting healthy eating. This is because Nature put our drugs in the food it provides, so we are to eat healthy to prevent diseases, heal diseases, and maintain good health.

In nutrition, you have to eat the right foods and avoid the wrong foods. Herbs also have to be used wisely. Some herbs interact with hypertension medications and shouldn't be used together.

A. Use of herbs

Garlic: This is one of the most popular and potent home remedies for treating high blood pressure. Garlic has many medicinal compounds and that is why it is used in treating a wide range of diseases including high blood pressure.

One of the strongest compounds in garlic that relieves high blood pressure is Allicin. However, it is unstable except it comes in contact with oxygen.

So, if you want to take garlic for therapeutic purposes, cut or crush few cloves of garlic and expose the cut or crushed garlic to air for few seconds and then you swallow them with a cup of warm water.

Do this at least once daily.

Coconut water: This is found inside the shell of green and unripe coconuts. In their raw and organic form, coconut water contains magnesium and potassium.

These minerals are needed for the control of muscle functions, including the heart which is a big and non-stop working muscle. Coconut water strengthens your heart to pump blood.

This reduces the pressure placed on the heart and also brings down high blood pressure. In studies, coconut water had a significant effect on systolic blood pressure.

This is the power that occurs when the heart pumps blood to all body parts. Drink 8 ounces of coconut water daily to benefit from this. Make sure you drink it in the morning when you wake up and also at night before you to bed.

Watermelon: Taking watermelon every morning before eating (on an empty stomach) is advised. It helps bring down high blood pressure. It contains an organic compound which is also an amino acid called Citrulline.

This amino acid is converted to L-arginine in the body when ingested. The body makes use of this to make nitric oxide, a compound that dilates the blood vessels.

Nitric oxide also regulates your vascular systemic resistance. This is how hard your heart pumps blood all through your whole body. It lowers vascular resistance by widening your blood vessels.

Have as many cups of fresh watermelon you can have daily. Eat more watermelon in the morning on an empty stomach. This would make it more effective.

Blueberry: Blueberry syrup is powerful in maintaining healthy blood pressure. This syrup here is a home-made type and not the ones produced commercially.

They are less healthy. Blueberries are rich in antioxidants, flavonoids, and Quercitin. These powerful nutrients dilate your blood vessels, improve the flow of blood and all these will help to put your blood pressure under control.

For this home-made syrup, you need the following:

- 8 cups of blueberries or you can mix it with elderberries. In this case, you need cups of blueberries and 4 cups of elderberries.
- A cup of raw honey
- 4 cups of clean water
- A glass jar with a good lid
- A strainer and a pot

Pour the dried berries and water in the pot and put it on a low heat and allow it to a simmer. Continue simmering until the liquid becomes half. Strain the liquid and pour the liquid back into the pot.

Add the honey and warm this mixture to make sure they mix thoroughly. Don't cook this syrup and make sure you get a slightly thin consistency.

Once you are done, store it in your glass jar and label. Keep it in the refrigerator for up to 4 weeks. Take a tablespoon of this twice daily.

Hibiscus tea: This is powerful in controlling blood pressure. It does this in many ways. First of all, it acts as a diuretic. This helps it draw sodium from the bloodstream.

This, in turn, would reduce the pressure on the walls of your arteries. Hibiscus also mimics the actions of angiotensin-converting enzyme (ACE) inhibitors.

ACE inhibitors are drugs used in treating high blood pressure. These drugs work by obstructing ACE and this compound carry out an important role in the renin-angiotensin system.

This is a hormone system that controls blood pressure and maintains the balance of fluids in the body. When this process is obstructed, the blood vessels relax, the blood volume is lowered, and the blood pressure also reduces.

Drink a cup of hibiscus tea two to three times daily. You can easily make this tea at home. Buy dried hibiscus leaves from the market and boil a good quantity of this.

You can boil it along with ginger, pineapple, or any other herb like lemongrass. You can also add lemon juice and honey to your hibiscus tea before drinking it.

Beetroots: These contain organic nitrates. The body uses this to make nitric oxide which is used in dilating your blood vessels. This would reduce blood pressure.

Blend whole beets and drink them without sieving. Take a glass of this juice three times daily.

Ginger: Ginger is one of the common and highly potent herbs used in treating high blood pressure naturally. It helps the smooth flow of blood in your body, thereby bring down high blood pressure.

Ginger can be taken alone or you can mix it with other herbs like cardamom, cinnamon, turmeric, lemon, Moringa, etc. Boil your fresh or dried ginger roots with any of the above-mentioned herbs.

You can also steep your ginger powder in a cup of boiling water for 10 minutes. Add lemon juice and raw honey to improve the taste of your ginger tea. Take a cup of this tea at least two times daily.

Basil: The leaves of Basil are rich in a compound called eugenol. This phytochemical prevent your blood vessels from constricting. It prevents them from becoming tight and blocked.

And all these causes blood pressure. A daily intake of this herb can relieve you of high blood pressure. Boil the leaves in water and drink this tea at least three times daily.

You can also add it generously to your meal. Other green leafy vegetables that reduce high blood pressure are spinach, celery, parsley, jute leaves, etc.

Hawthorn: This is a heart-healthy herb. It contains a high amount of Quercitin and flavonoids, especially oligomeric procyanidins (OPC's). Flavonoids have a lot of amazing health benefits but the most studied aspect is the benefit of flavonoids on heart disease.

Untreated or uncontrolled hypertension leads to heart disease. Hawthorn relieves the symptoms of arrhythmia, it improves the functions of your blood vessels, relieves palpitations, regulates the metabolism of glucose, reduces arterial blood pressure, and also lowers your risks of hypertension and heart disease.

Flavonoids expand your blood vessels and this, in turn, lower blood pressure. You can drink hawthorn tea daily or take them in the form of "balls" since it is a rich source of flavonoids.

To make hawthorn balls, you need the following:

- 4 tablespoons of hawthorn berry
- 1 tablespoon of ginger and cinnamon each. They improve the circulation of blood in the body.
- Carob powder or cocoa powder
- Water and raw honey

Pour the ginger powder, cinnamon, and hawthorn in a small bowl and mix these ingredients. Add enough water and raw honey until it forms a thick paste.

You can thicken it with cocoa or carob powder. Mix properly until it forms into a dough. Roll this dough into clean balls. The balls should not be bigger than your index fingernails.

Arrange these balls on a cookie sheet and dry them in an oven using a very low temperature. The temperature should not be more than 1500F. Make sure they are well dried.

Store these balls indefinitely in a glass jar with a good tight lid. Keep this jar in a cool dry place and out of direct sunlight. Eat a good quantity of these daily.

Cat's claw: For thousands of years, this herb has been used as a traditional remedy for a lot of ailments including hypertension. It dilates the blood vessels and boosts the flow of blood all through the body.

This helps to lower blood pressure. It also acts as a diuretic because it contains tannins and flavonoids. It gets rid of excess salt and water thereby reducing high blood pressure.

A decoction of cat's claw is usually given to patients with high blood pressure. A decoction is the same as tea but in this case, it is simmered for a longer time and it is the woody and tough parts of the plants like the steam, barks, or roots that are used.

Pregnant women should avoid this herb. Pour 2 tablespoons of this herb and a cup of water in a pot. Reduce the heat and leave it to simmer for 40 to 45 minutes.

Depending on how thick you want it to be, you can add more water or less.

Strain and add lemon or honey or both.
Drink this decoction once daily.

B. Nutrition

Avoid salt: Sodium, one of the chemical components of salt is not good for people with high blood pressure. Excess sodium would disrupt the balance of fluid in your body.

In a bid to remove excess sodium from your body, excess water will be drawn from surrounding tissues to expel the salt. This volume accumulates more in your heart.

This would increase the pressure on your heart and make it harder to pump blood. So avoid table salts and canned and processed foods. These foods contain high levels of salt.

You need the power of will to do this. Note that there is a high amount of sodium in processed and canned foods. So, avoid these and junks also.

Avoid caffeine and alcohol: Even in little amounts, alcohol raises your blood pressure. Excess of it will make it difficult to control your blood pressure.

Healthy people can take moderate amounts of caffeine but hypertensive patients should avoid it. It makes blood pressure difficult to control in hypertensive patients.

Avoid processed meats: These are made by soaking them in a brine bath made of spices and salt.

Avoid white bread, butter, and margarine: All these are loaded with salts and fats that are not good for you. They increase your levels of cholesterol and this can worsen hypertension and even lead to heart disease.

Avoid refined sugars: These make your arteries expand at a fast rate. When this continues happening, your arteries would become fragile and weak.

This will lead to high blood pressure and also make your arteries prone to rupture. When this happens, cholesterol/plaque will attach itself to the damaged artery thereby reducing the flow of blood and increasing your blood pressure.

C. Hydrotherapy

Hydrotherapy is the act of healing with water. Water can be used to dilate your blood vessels. In hydrotherapy, water is used to reduce the overdrive from the sympathetic nervous system.

Hydrotherapy is also used to excrete sodium and excess water. There are many ways hydrotherapists reduce high blood pressure.

1. By Drinking: They encourage their patients to increase their intake of water. This would prevent dehydration which worsens hypertension.

Your body is constantly drawing water to eliminate excess sodium and other toxins in your body. You have to take in clean water. Ensure that you are properly hydrated.

Water also helps in the elimination of toxins, wastes, and excess sodium in the body. Toxicity is a risk factor for high blood pressure. Excess sodium and wastes products in the body also lead to hypertension.

Warm or hot water is ideal for this. You can also drink lukewarm water. However, cold water is discouraged because it constricts your blood vessels instead of dilating them.

This would worsen hypertension and increase the symptoms.

2. A hot foot bath and fomentation placed over the flanks: More than 40% of hypertensive patients have a high content of sodium. Their bodies retain a high amount of sodium.

Hypertensive patients are also sensitive to sodium. Physiologically, anywhere you find sodium, you would find water. If the excess amount of sodium in your body is not excreted through the kidneys (urine), it would stay in your blood and increase the volume of your blood.

This, in turn, would lead to high blood pressure. A diuretic can aid the expulsion of excess sodium from the body. It makes it easy for the kidneys to expel a high amount of salt and water.

This process can be added by having a hot foot bath. Then a hot fomentation is placed over the kidneys for 20 minutes. This is done two times daily. This will improve the production and output of urine. This will also improve the flow of blood to the kidneys.

Avoid things that reduce the flow of blood to the kidneys such as the wrong diets. Anything that reduces blood flow to your kidneys will increase your blood pressure.

Even though should be done by a hydrotherapist, you can do it yourself.

Just stick to the rules. Do not exceed 20 minutes and it should be done not more than two times daily.

A fomentation is the act of apply warm, hot, soft, or medicinal substances on your skin to relieve pain, relax the skin, or disperse tumors. In this case, you can put hot water in a bottle and close it tight.

Place this bottle on your kidneys. You can also use a clean towel soaked in hot water. Remember to drink water to help the process of eliminating sodium.

3. General revulsive hydrotherapy consisting of a hot foot bath, cold compress to the head, fomentation to the spine, and alternate hot and cold bath to the abdomen: All these would help to reduce high blood pressure.

Heat to the spinal cord will calm the overactive sympathetic nerves. This, in turn, would improve the flow of blood to your kidneys.

4. Neural tube bath: This involves soaking in water that has a temperature of 94 to 97 degrees Fahrenheit. This will relax your body and reduce your blood pressure.

This will also help to calm your overactive sympathetic nervous system.

Contraindications

Hypertensive patients should not undergo hot baths, steam baths, and saunas. They all lead to massive vasodilation and the individual will faint.

Patients taking vasodilators should not be given any heating treatment.

D. Aromatherapy

Aromatherapy is the act of inhaling scents of essential oils to treat health conditions. Essential oils are gotten from medicinal plants and they contain the healing compound of the plant they were gotten from in concentrated amounts.

They can be massage on the skin when diluted and they can also be inhaled. Inhaling these medicinal plants are known to correct a lot of health problems like high blood pressure.

You can use a blend or mixture of the following oils: Neroli, ylang-ylang, marjoram, and lavender. Diffuse this blend in your home using a diffuser or just add 2 drops of this oil to your handkerchief and keep inhaling it.

You can also take in this oil but you have to check with a naturopath to be safe. Some essential oils are not safe for consumption, some must be diluted before consuming, and some might react with your drugs.

Essential oils that have been studied and known to have a therapeutic effect on blood pressure are:

Ylang ylang

Yarrow

Valerian

Sweet marjoram

Sage

Rose

Neroli

Lime

Lemon balm

Lemon

Lavender

Helichrysum

Jasmine

Frankincense

Clary sage

Citronella

Cedarwood

Bergamot

Remember that these oils have very concentrated amounts of the healing components of the plants they were extracted from. So you have to use them with care.

You can dilute them and also massage your body with the blend. It will also help regulate your blood pressure. `

E. Heliotherapy

Heliotherapy is the art of healing with sunlight. Sunlight helps you maintain healthy blood pressure. It also helps correct high blood pressure. Sunlight does this in many ways.

Nitric oxide is present on the top layer of your skin. When you expose yourself to sunlight, this nitric oxide will react with the healing rays of the sun and dilate your blood vessels.

This act widens your blood vessels, normalizes the flow of blood, and restores your blood pressure to normal. Many people don't know that the skin is involved in the regulation of blood pressure and this depends on your exposure to gentle sunlight.

Another way sunlight regulates your blood pressure is by increasing your level of vitamin D. This important vitamin/hormone restores your body to its natural balance.

This includes the regulation of blood pressure.

Now, scientists are looking for ways to use ultraviolet light in the treatment of high blood pressure and heart disease. To benefit from this, you have to sunbathe daily.

Expose yourself to the gentle rays of sunrise and sunset daily. Do not wear sunscreen or use other forms of sunblock. Avoid intense sunlight. You can also practise sun gazing. It will improve your overall health.

F. Exercise

This is another effective way to lower your blood pressure naturally. Sedentary people have high risks of hypertension than active people.

Regular exercise would empower your heart to pump more blood. This would reduce the pressure on your heart and the force on your arteries. This, in turn, would bring down high blood pressure.

Aerobic exercises are ideal for your blood pressure and overall health. This includes walking, cycling, jogging, dancing, swimming, bicycling, climbing stairs, and active sports like tennis, football, or basketball.

This exercise also includes house chores like gardening, mowing the lawn, scrubbing the floor, raking leaves, and doing your laundry. The idea behind this is just to move your body.

You don't need to spend hours in the gym every day. Just making your daily life active and full of activities can give you this benefit. This simply means that you have to make little changes to your daily routine to benefit from exercise.

Set time for walking or other exercises of your choice. Be more engaged in house chores. Engage in exercise or physical activities that increase your breathing rate and heartbeat.

Short exercises that last for at least 10 minutes are better than no exercise at all.

Conclusion

Simple activities can turn you into a healthy human being in no time. You just have to remember that you cannot overstress. You have to make a plan to perform one time exercise every day, eat good food, and watch your habits. Being less stressed about your condition is another way of solving the problem. Since mental stress is a major cause of high blood pressure, you have to seek easier ways of doing things and only do things that will favor your stress-free endeavor henceforth.

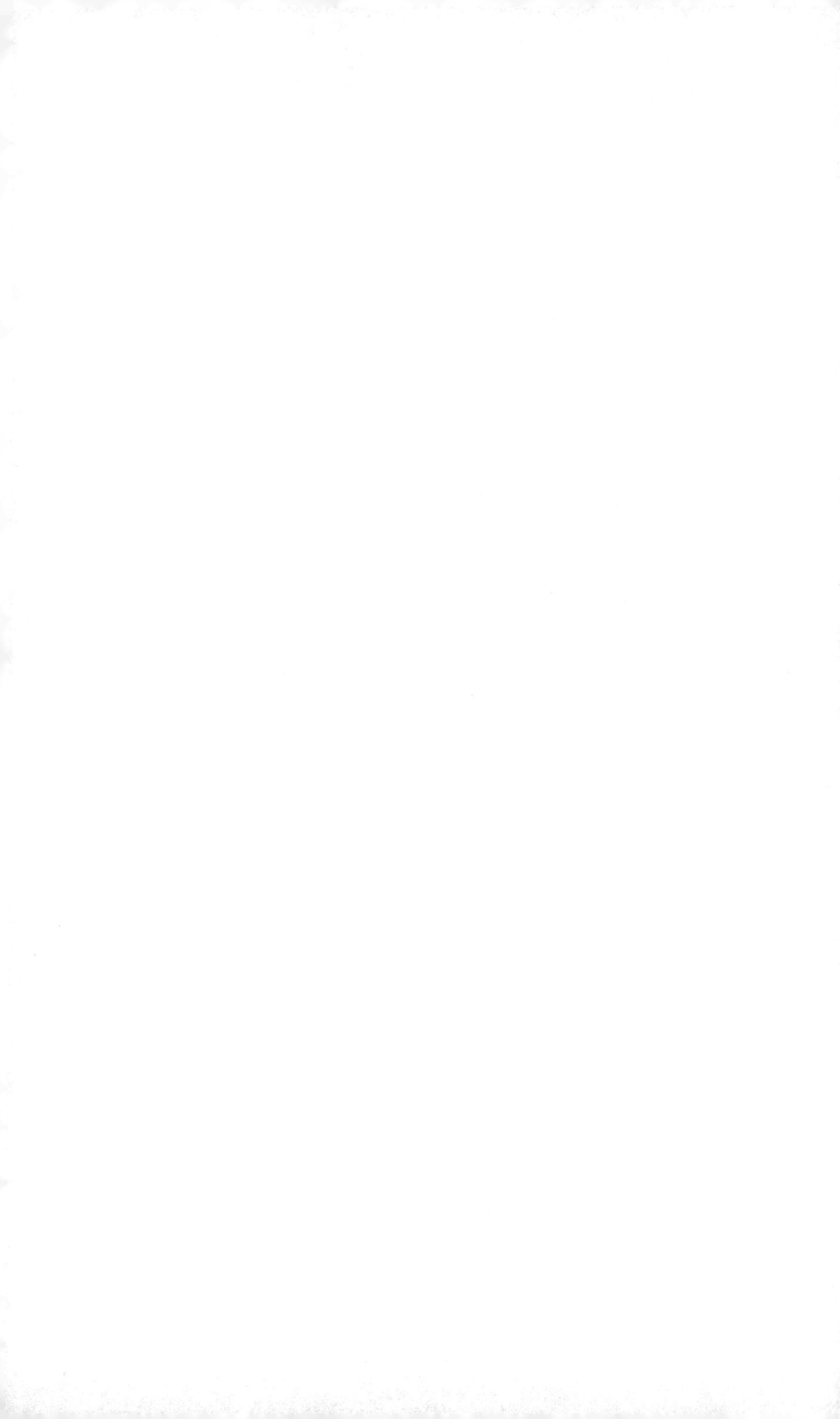

9 781980 491040